Travel Physical Therapy For New Graduates

How I Paid off $83,000 of Student Loans in Under 1.5 Years

Dr. Matthew Del Tufo PT, DPT

Table of Contents

Introduction:

Welcome new graduates to the world of travel therapy. I am writing this book because this was the career path that I never learned about in school, and one that I never even knew existed until a chance meeting during my third and final clinical rotation just prior to graduation. I have made a career out of being a traveling physical therapist since graduation and, simply put, it has been the best career decision I could have made for a plethora of reasons. Following this path has allowed me to travel the country, become completely debt free from my sizeable student loans, and gain a much more diverse clinical skill set than I could have ever hoped to build in a permanent job setting. I did all of this, and much more, in less than two years. This was all completed without any guidance or trailblazers in front of me who could point me to the starting line, tell me what to expect from this career path, or exactly how this unique job market worked. I had to discover the ins and outs of this business myself, and in doing so made just about every mistake out there. I was forced to learn while on the job, which became a constant process of failing forward over and over again. This caused me to lose out on quite a bit financially during my first year of this journey and unfortunately made things much harder than they could, or should have been. This book is designed to save you from the shortcomings I experienced, and supply you with all the information I wish I had when starting on this incredible journey. In short this is the travel therapy blueprint for new graduates. This book will provide you with step-by-step directions to take you all the way from passing your boards, to landing your first contract, and beyond.

This book is broken down into three distinct sections to make things as easy as possible to take in. It is a clear and concise format with every section providing a unique purpose. Part one will tell you about the traveling healthcare profession. It will give you information on how it works, what it is, and will shed an honest light on the benefits and drawbacks of the business. Part two will take you through my story from graduating, and passing the boards to accepting my first contract. It will show you exactly what my starting position was, and very likely demonstrate how comparable yours is to it now. Part three is what you really came here for, as it is the actual blueprint that needs to be followed. It will inform you on the best ways to go about choosing a company that is right for you, interviewing for contracts, what you absolutely need to have written in a contract, and getting you to the location along with much more. It is the part of the book that will literally save you thousands of dollars that I missed out on, but you will not. Enjoy the journey my friends and colleagues, I hope to meet you on the road.

- Dr. Matthew Del Tufo PT, DPT

"A ship in harbor is safe, but that is not what ships are made for"
- John A. Shedd

Part One: The Traveling Therapist Profession

Understanding the Traveling Healthcare Provider Profession:

A traveling healthcare provider is someone who works on a contract-to-contract basis without any long-term commitments. Contracts can be found from as little as four weeks all the way up to a full year, but by far the most available and commonly seen come in packages of thirteen and twenty-six weeks. Now as a physical therapist these assignments are in various settings including private or hospital based outpatient practices, all inpatient hospital settings, home health opportunities, as well as skilled nursing facilities. This availability may change depending on your profession whether it be occupational therapy, speech therapy, or nursing. Not only are the potential range of settings numerous, but so is the availability of locations to choose from. Contracts for traveling healthcare providers exist in every state across the nation without exception, which is consequently one of the main driving factors for those participating in this profession. Have you ever wanted to live in the mountains in Colorado? What about the rocky coastlines of Oregon, or sunny California, how about the big island of Hawaii? The possibilities and experiences are literally endless, which allows you to create your own unique path through life. This variety and flexibility that you are offered to choose from is unmatched by just about any other career opportunity and truly gives you an unreal balance of work and play. For me travel healthcare lets me live a life of adventure while sharpening my clinical skill set as a physical therapist, all the while providing greater pay than I could receive elsewhere as a new graduate.

Now we can answer one of the most commonly asked questions relating to our profession:

"Why would a facility or a company need a traveler or contract worker for their business?"

This can be due to a wide variety of reasons, but the most common I have found to be true through my years of traveling include:
- Seasonal environments where, for example, populations surge in the summers and thus deliver a very high census for a short period of time
- Maternity leave
- Current therapists leaving a company for a new job creating extended absences
- Expanding and growing private practices
- Clinics may prefer travelers because it simply makes more financial sense for them i.e. They do not have to provide health insurance
- A clinic may be having difficulty hiring permanent staff due to location or other various reasons

I am confident that there are many other reasons from a business perspective, but these are the ones I notice to repeat over and over again. Another thing you may very well find is that clinics that utilize travelers seldom do it once. As one traveler's contract is ending they will either offer an extension, or hire a new one to pick up where they left off to minimize lapses in service. This is good for our profession as it provides a fresh rotation of jobs to choose from in the market.

What are the drawbacks to being a traveler?

While travel therapy is really a great gig, and one that is hard to beat in terms of its overall flexibility and financial incentives it is still not without its drawbacks. Some of these drawbacks may vary somewhat person to person and may be more applicable to an individual depending on various aspects including what their company may assist or entirely take care of for them. Regardless this list will give you a good idea of potential job annoyances that you are likely to experience.

1. The pre-assignment paperwork: In the travel world the work begins before you ever get to your new assignment's location. This prerequisite list can range from short and quick to a rather lengthy list that may leave you scratching your head as to how on earth will I get all this done. This is largely determined by where you will be working and in what setting you will be working in. For example hospitals can be very

strict requiring multiple tests, verifications, and other hoops to jump through before you ever set foot in the door while a private practices just might be looking to make sure you have a state license and that your CPR/AED certification is up to date. Pre-assignment work can commonly include tumultuous paperwork that you will need to wade through, various blood tests, drug tests, TB tests, immunization records, background checks, CPR/AED certification proof, and fingerprinting. Paperwork is never fun regardless of career and traveling healthcare is no exception. Luckily almost everything you complete as a prerequisite for one assignment will apply to future contracts. A good example would again be your CPR/AED certification, which may be good for 2 years, or a TB test completed in the same calendar year. It does force you to keep neat records for yourself as well, but your company will keep these documents on file to streamline the process for you and get you working quickly.

2. Getting licensed: I am going to speak on this one from a physical therapist's perspective as the laws and regulations may be different for occupational therapists or speech therapists, etc. As of now if you are a PT licensed in one state and want to work in another you will have to acquire that state's license to be eligible. Now this may be changing shortly due to the current landscape and the soon to be enacted compact via the FSBPT. This new compact, which is to go into effect sometime in the second half of 2018 will allow you to work in any state that is

involved through compact privilege. Exactly how this works has not yet been made clear, but it is a great thing for any new traveling Physical Therapists and will make life that much easier. Since it is not yet enacted I will tell you getting licensed in various states you would like to work in is an essential nuisance that all will go through. Getting licenses generally requires time to get the application ready, pass any jurisprudence exam if applicable, obtain verifications from other states in which you are licensed, and complete any other unique requirements before returning all of this information to a state's professional board. If there is a state you know you want to work in then your best course of action is to begin the application process early. Most travelers will begin one license while still working a previous contract. This is to ensure that when their current contract ends the new license will be issued making them ready and able to begin working immediately if they so choose. This can be a headache with the severity of the ensuing headache being completely dependent on where you want to go. For example, Oregon is an awesome state that had me licensed and ready to work within two weeks. California, on the other hand, had taken three months after I had submitted all the required material.

3. Packing Stress: This one will affect all individuals differently. As a traveler you are essentially forced to travel lightly. Realistically you have as much space as is available in your car and no more. This can create packing stress

for many as you are deciding what to leave, and what to bring with you to your new location. I have discussed this topic extensively with many travelers and all have different approaches and priorities. Your packing list may include clothes, personal items, kitchen or laundry matter, fitness equipment, small pieces of furniture, air mattresses, and sporting equipment such as golf clubs or snowboards amongst other things. It is up to you in deciding what you really need and what belongings you can either survive without or pick up along the way. You also have to remember that when you are taking 13-week contracts you must be ready and able to pack up and move your life all over again in very short order. For some this is harder than others, but it is something all travelers quickly become accustomed to. In most situations you will enjoy the simplicity of owning less while discovering what the real necessary items are, and the others you only thought were.

4. Housing: Finding housing can often be anxiety inducing to many in the traveling world. No one is truly immune to the concerns caused by this step. This is because you are moving to a brand new area, with little to no knowledge of it except where you will be working. Not only that you are assigned the task of finding short term, safe, and suitable housing. You can always let your company do this step for you, but every traveler I have ever met, including myself, will highly recommend taking the stipend and completing this step yourself for reasons we will get into later in the book. While this is a worry with

every new assignment you take, it is one that always seems to turn out fine one way or another. Through apartment complexes, to online social media groups, and other websites this step has become easier and will soon become a skill like any other that you will develop as you travel.

5. The lonely road: New graduates will, in due course, get used to the idea of road tripping to a new location, and then beginning their contract independently. In the early stages when following this career path it can cause a bit of apprehension and even fear. So the age-old question of, do travelers get lonely? The answer is yes, but only sometimes. Road tripping alone, and moving into your apartment alone can make you feel isolated at times, but there are plenty of ways to meet people and find new friends as you arrive in an area. Often times your new social circle may come in the form of coworkers, while in other situations it may be new friends you meet at the gym or out in town. I have never arrived in a new location and failed to make friends within the first week or two. There are also a multitude of apps and online social media groups to find new people so you will undoubtedly locate those who have similar areas of interest, or hobbies as you no matter where you go.

6. The workload: This was a concern I had when beginning traveling as many professors who discouraged me from this profession told me horror stories of travelers being taken advantage

of in the workplace. I have again, and again found this not to be true. My caseload is always the same or closely in line with all others who work at a given clinic. What you do need to realize as a traveler is that you are expected to be able to adapt quickly to your new environment, and become independent in short order. This is not a clinical rotation in the sense that you have a mentor in place that will slow walk you around until you are comfortable. As a traveler you will first have an orientation that is often short lived. Following this you typically will get a quick facility tour, meet some of the staff who are currently available, and given a brief overview of the documentation system. It is worth pointing out that learning the new documenting system is typically the biggest hassle we all face when arriving at a new clinic. Every time you take a new contract expect to begin with a brand new system that you have yet to encounter. You will then begin seeing your patients within a day or two to begin building your caseload, which means if you are not quick on your feet it is possible to fall behind with your schedule and paperwork early on. Many new travelers can be blindsided by this aspect, but this will be less of a concern if you follow the blueprint in section 3 for navigating the phone interview. In doing so you will know exactly what to expect on arrival including orientation time, and much more.

The above list encompasses many of the negative aspects of being a traveler, but do not be afraid. There are numerous benefits to being a traveling healthcare worker that I can now speak of from my own personal experience. From professional growth as a therapist and financial gain, to adventure and exploration it is a career that is truly unmatched. I'll give you just a taste of some of the good life through this short section.

First and foremost you get to travel and live in a whole new area for three months at a time! I have found this to be the perfect amount of time to really explore an area without things becoming stale or repetitive. Throughout the assignment you will be working during the week, and likely staying nearby your work office or housing area. It is here where you will meet many people from the community and make some new friends whether it be from work, the gym, or just on some nights out. Once the weekend comes you can make your plans to explore the surrounding areas and see what your new location really has to offer. Where you adventure to will depend entirely on what you are looking for. For one person it may be outdoor activities such as hiking in nearby parks or camping. For others it may be exploring cities that have their own unique attractions and sights. There are a lot of possibilities and given the length of an assignment that gives you thirteen potential weekends for adventures. Even the areas that do not seem to have a lot of activities nearby will be able to provide fun new experiences to fill an itinerary for each weekend. I personally am looking for contracts that are in close proximity to national parks, beaches, or bigger cities that I have yet to visit. These are my interests, but by choosing a contract in a new area that is desirable to you will provide you with plenty of fun for your short time visiting.

A second great benefit of working as a traveling healthcare provider is the variety of clinical skills you will pick up. I can happily say that through travel I have grown more professionally far more than I ever could have hoped to in a permanent job setting. This is solely due to the vast number of new physical therapists I am constantly exposed to on a routine basis. Each new contract brings me to new clinics where people have different skill sets and specialties. This ranges from advanced manual certifications, population specific techniques, and new ways of problem solving difficult cases. This was, and still is, great for me because as a new graduate trying to make my way in this profession I only had the tools that were picked up at school plus clinical rotations. While these skills were sufficient to begin the process of treating patients, and working successfully as a physical therapist I found myself quick to realize there is more learning to be done. Watching and experiencing more seasoned therapists first hand has allowed me to pick up on new methods that I could then apply to my own practice. This has also allowed me to see the benefits of certain advanced credentials in practice that I may wish to pursue in the near future. It also displayed the exact opposite in specific situations where techniques I may have initially thought were useful are not as applicable, and do not have the evidence or outcomes needed for me to pursue them professionally.

While traveling the country to explore new landscapes and experience new places while improving clinical skills in the real world are both huge benefits of this profession there is still the elephant in the room I have yet to mention. Working as a traveling healthcare provider is undoubtedly the most impactful way to change your financial situation. This is even more pronounced as a new graduate when you are beginning your career search with no experience, and tons of student loan debt that will be picking up interest in the impending months. Every company you interview with will happily pay you less as a new graduate, but this does not have to be the case. Due to the way I started my career as a traveler I went from fresh out of school to making more money than the majority of private practice owners. Working as a traveler just turned the least financially productive years of my working career to potentially the highest I may ever experience. Let us do a quick runaround of the finances so I may tell you how this is possible. First, as a traveler you get paid an hourly wage which like any job is taxed. The amount you earn may be the same, or slightly less than the market average in your given area. Next you will receive a housing stipend that is based on GSA rates by the government for the area you will be working in. This money is not taxable and is given to provide living conditions for the length of your contract. Finally you will receive a food stipend that is also based on GSA rates. As you can guess this is also not taxable and is used for your food expenses while on assignment. With both stipends what is not used for its designated purposes is simply yours to keep! This is a big deal period. It is also the real deciding factor that influenced me to give travel therapy a shot despite not knowing a thing about it and having no one to guide me through the process. As all new graduates know the student debt and loan crisis is a real thing. Once you are out of school and real life begins you quickly see how it will impact all financial decisions going forward. By choosing this career I have proudly paid off all of my student loans from graduate school, $83,000+ in total, within one year and four months of work, and I am telling you it is possible for you as well.

Is this career really for new graduates?

This is a tough question that everyone will have to decide for him or herself. I have gone over several of the larger positive and negative aspects of this career path so that you may have an idea of what you are getting yourself into, which is much more than I had going in. I will give you my honest answer to the question though. Yes, simply yes! I think this is not only a viable option for any new graduate who just received their diploma, but also the best option. The vast majority of us who are fresh out of school are somewhere in our 20's or maybe early 30's. This is a great time in your life to travel, and it may also be the only time you can do so in such a way until you are retired. You can explore the country right now while you are strong, able bodied, and still adventurous enough to do it.

This becomes less and less likely as you form more serious relationships, have children, and begin to accumulate other ties to an area or community. Through your travels you may even find a new area that you would like to live in, or a permanent home and workplace through one of your contracts. This career will not only make you a better healthcare provider, but it will expand your professional network nationwide. You will become much more financially stable in the process as it situates you in a more advantageous position to tackle your student loans and begin building wealth. My advice to any new graduate who asks me what to do is to take the first two years out of school, and pursue life as a traveling therapist. You should use the money you make to free yourself from student loans, and the experience of traveling to create memories and stories that you will have for the rest of your life. In the absolute worst-case scenario you may try this path and decide after your first thirteen-week contract that it is not for you. You can stop then and there as there is no obligation to anything after that first contract. You can stop, go home, pick up a permanent job, and resume your previous life knowing that you gave it an honest go.

Part Two: My Story

I want to give you a brief background of myself, and how I began my journey from graduating from physical therapy school with my doctorate in hand, passing the boards, and getting started as a traveling physical therapist. I want to do this for several reasons. One is so you can understand how little I actually knew about this profession when I first began. Another reason is that it will give you an honest assessment of your starting position compared to mine, and likely how similar they really are. I think this section is also important because getting started on any path is often the hardest part, and this is never truer then when you are finally beginning your career fresh off graduation. Doing so without guidance, knowing what to expect, and with a seemingly insurmountable amount of student loan debt at your side just adds to an already difficult decision. This section is to help you deal with the uncertainties that everyone faces, and will demonstrate how it all works in a realistic perspective.

We are going to begin this story when I was in my third and final year of graduate school completing the final clinical rotation. It was during this rotation that I had a chance meeting that, unbeknownst to me at the time, would change my whole career path. Not only that it would greatly alter where I would live, and work for the next two years and counting.

My first encounter with anyone in the traveling healthcare profession came roughly midway through that final rotation. It was a normal day for me coming into the clinic, looking at my caseload, and eyeing up the amount of work put before me that day, but all of a sudden I noticed a new face at one of the desks. At this time I was pretty familiar with all my coworkers so when I saw a new woman I assumed she was a new hire or potentially another student? I was wrong. I asked my CI if they had just hired anyone, but he promptly told me she was a contract worker that their hospital uses from time to time. I did not fully grasp what he meant and just assumed he was referring to a per diem kind of deal as we carried on with our day. I started becoming more interested as other workers started referring to her as the new traveler, which of course did not make any sense to me as to why you would call a new per diem worker that. It eventually happened enough times to the point where I was curious enough to ask her about it and what they meant.

That began one of our many conversations about her career path, and of course where I first learned that a traveling physical therapist was an actual thing. Not only was she generous with her time answering my abundant questions, but also she gave me glimpses into the inner workings of how contract professionals worked. This made me quick to realize how great of a career path this could potentially be. Over the next weeks I began talking to her more and more, slowly prying into her life and career. She was incredibly helpful, and not shy at all in discussing her previous jobs across several different states. I was shown the different clinics she worked at, pictures from road trips, and much more. I took in as much information as I could in while she filled in the gaps including the basics of how it worked, how she found housing while on assignments, and of course more pictures of her adventures that instantly made me incredibly jealous. I used all the free time I had to learn what I could from her, but all too soon my final weeks were winding down, and I was back in class to finish up the remainder of the semester where I would finally graduate from PT school.

Back in school now with the semester wrapping up I, unfortunately, began letting the memories and excitement from the conversations I had with the traveling therapist slip from my mind. I believe a lot of this was due to the way our professors' and physical therapy program presented life after graduation to us. It put everyone in our cohort, more or less, on the same route that would go something like: make your walk for graduation to mark the end of school, take and pass your boards, search for jobs that are within commuting distance from your home to limit costs, interview in the setting you found most enjoyable throughout your clinical rotations, and begin working. That may sound familiar to a lot of you reading this book as the traditional path. After completing those steps you then are supposed to continue progressing your skills as a PT, get an advanced certification or two, and that is essentially your life for the next forty years until you reach retirement. That is what we all are supposed to do right? Well that is what I thought anyway, and I am sure many of you reading this have come to the same conclusion. Between talking to my professors, and hearing what my classmates had to say it seemed like the only option.

I almost resigned myself to this life plan as I had some semblance of an idea of which settings I was more interested in working, but was still was not one hundred percent certain I wanted it for a full time job for the next forty plus years. There were also quite a few uncertainties I felt that were never fully addressed in school, which left us all in the dark on several important aspects of life that were about to be thrust upon us as we enter the real world. One of the main ones of course was how much should we expect to make as a new graduate coming straight out of school? Salary, or any financial information for that matter, felt like a taboo subject through our curriculum. As if there was some form of a nonverbal agreement that made it a forbidden topic that was not to be discussed openly in class. This subject became of ever-increasing importance to our class as we were coming into graduation, which was likely the result of seeing the total amount of student loan debt we would all be leaving school with. Others were also thinking about the further real world possibilities of starting families, and buying cars or houses. All of that crucial life responsibilities that was put to the side while in school was about to come crashing to the forefront leaving only a hazy picture of what was next for us. My mind at this time was transitioning from, "I hope I passed that last practical," to, "I hope I am not in debt forever because of this!"

We were in the final two weeks of classes when I finally began to remember the traveling therapist I met while on clinical, and how excited she seemed to be on a constant vacation with new places to explore while in sound financial space. It was on my mind so much I decided it necessary to begin seeking advice from the faculty in regards to that career path. I started tracking them down one by one during their office hours to discover if they knew of any traveling therapists personally, including prior students, who have gone through with this career path, and for their personal thoughts if this was an advisable decision for a new graduate. I can say while I went into all of these impromptu meetings with high optimism, I often left them, to my dismay, discouraged to say the least. The vast majority stated that this was not a good plan and most certainly not for new graduates. The closest thing I got to a positive notion of this career path went something along the lines of; you should take a job to build experience and find your groove, and then after one to three years of work if you are still interested begin researching it. The idea of waiting years on a potential career opportunity that was available now just did not appeal to me. To me this meant starting out as a new grad in a new clinic with no experience and thusly receiving a lower salary, getting comfortable in an area and workplace environment that would likely make it more difficult to leave your stable position, and continuing to be in substantial debt from graduate school.

I ended up discussing my lofty ideas with one more professor who provided me with the same disappointing story informing me that this was likely not a suitable position for new graduates, and then threw in an extra horror story of travelers being taken advantage of for good measure. I remember this next part very clearly as I was about to resign myself to the traditional route described above upon passing my boards. I left the office and walked down the stairs and sat on a bench out in the sun. There was about an hour to go before our next class so I had some time to kill. I pulled out my phone, and got on social media to find a few traveling companies whose names I had remembered from past research. I found a number and without much thought gave them a call.

Before I knew it a delightful woman picked up the phone, and we chatted for a bit while I asked her a ridiculous number of questions. I told her my story of where I was currently located, how much of the school year was left and the upcoming graduation date, when I was planning on taking the boards, and if all goes well where I will be licensed. She began telling me about the profession, some of the details of it, and about their company. I remember asking her my biggest concern at the time, which was if this was a suitable career for new graduates, or if they only worked with more experienced therapists. She promptly laughed telling me they have worked with individuals of all kinds of experience. This included new grads that want to work full time to those with 20+ years experience who only want to work a few days a week. This conversation was a big turning point for me as it was when I knew I was not going to listen to the dissuading council I had previously received, but instead follow my own route. It gave me faith that this idea was not so out there after all, and has been done countless times before. After answering several more of my questions leaving me wishing I had planned the phone call better to actually write down her answers, the woman took down my number and email so that we would keep in touch. She told me they would stay in contact while I focused on passing the board's exam so that we could then begin looking for my first assignment afterward. With my mind at ease I was ready to finish up what remained of the semester. I thought it was going to be smooth sailing from here, but unfortunately there were still several obstacles that I would have to overcome.

With a quick fast forward school was over, I had made my walk for graduation, and was now studying for the boards. I was studying while working that summer as an ocean lifeguard, which was the only other meaningful job I have had since I was 16 years old. I hit the books after work every day for an hour or two reading the Scorebuilders textbook and taking the practice exams. Combine that with the PEAT practice exams I passed the boards very comfortably on my first attempt in July. The woman I talked to from the traveling company had been true to her word and stayed in contact with me through the whole process. We communicated by email and texts about once every two or three weeks as she was checking in to see how my studying was going. Once I found out I passed the boards I immediately let her know and we began having more serious talks about potential assignments and where I would like to start looking for jobs. Despite going to school in New Jersey I was initially licensed in Virginia so that is where we started.

The process began nicely and had an initial easy flow to all of it. I gave a potential start date for the end of summer when the beaches close and lifeguarding for me would come to an end. I was promptly emailed a list of potential assignments with the location and setting for which I would be working in. I picked out several assignments I may be interested in and sent my choices back so that I may be submitted for interviews. At the time I was thinking that this was going to be an easy walk in the park. I thought I would just hang back and let the interviews and job offers come to me, but unfortunately this is not what ended up happening. Now before going forward I want to point out that this is the period where I discovered that some of the locations for travel assignments given to me were way out in the middle of nowhere, which is a very common occurrence for travel jobs. The opportunities in more desirable locations are posted and gone in a day. This is a fast business, and you have to be ready to move on the contracts when they are offered.

It turned out that getting the first contract was more difficult than I originally anticipated. I went into this a little naive and expected to pick up a contract and begin working pretty quickly. For my first assignment this was not true as I had applied for at least six assignments and was still without an interview. Anytime I asked for updates the company and woman I was working with at the time would inform me that they were either waiting for a reply, had already chosen someone with more experience, or total radio silence. This went on for two more weeks and I was getting a bit frustrated with the process and worried at the same time that this idea of a career would not work out. It became enough of a concern that when I was offered an interview for a permanent job an hour from my home I took it thinking I should hear out all of my options.

My first interview for a permanent position was with an outpatient private practice, and honestly it went great. The facility was up to date with brand new equipment, the caseload seemed manageable although a bit on the high end, and that famous line of there is ample room to grow and move up in the company was used. Here are the real details and numbers from that interview. I was initially offered $68,000 starting salary as a new graduate with a $2,500 bonus after the first year. Every year they do an evaluation and you will get a small percentage raise. They also offered 2 weeks of paid vacation, and a pretty good health coverage plan. It was nothing great all things considered, but it was reasonable offer and a safe bet. I could tell my parents, who never interfere in my life decisions, definitely liked that idea over my only slightly thought out travel plans. The interview took place on a Thursday and was told they would like to have my answer by Monday.

After struggling with the initial travel company I was working with I decided to contact a second one. There are many companies out there and I was essentially deciding on who to contact through their website design and social media presence, which is definitely not how I recommend to go about this now. I called the second company on the same day after being offered the permanent position. This was a company with fewer overall reviews from what I could find scouring the Internet, however the several I managed to dig up were largely positive. Another woman answered the phone when I called and we went through a similar process as I did with the first company. We talked about my recent graduation and passing the boards as well as which states I was licensed in and where I would be interested in working. I had them send me an available job list, but then they also did something different. They discussed with me that many assignments are looking for more experienced workers however there are still quite a few specific facilities they had used in the past that were more open to new graduates. I was asked my opinion regarding several other states with shorter licensing timelines to comply with my tentative start date, and they got to work. Before I knew it I had my first interview lined up for Saturday morning and the ball was moving again.

Saturday arrived and since I was working I had my first interview as a traveler on the beach in board shorts while lifeguarding. I was told beforehand via email what time I would be called, the person's name who would be calling, the pay package being offered, and a little bit of information about the facility so I could plan accordingly. Looking back I had no idea what I was doing or how this interview process worked besides the fact that it was a phone interview. I did not have any questions written down, did not know was important to ask, and the overall idea was to wing it and feel things out as the conversation unfolded.

My phone rang right on schedule and the interview began. It felt like a whirlwind and before I knew it, maybe fifteen whole minutes later the whole thing was done. I will say I got lucky in this interview because the woman conducting it was very thorough. She spent the majority of the time telling me about the facility, the daily schedule, what was expected of me, along with a long list of information that I likely should have been writing down. At the end she asked what I thought and if I had any questions. I felt obligated to ask something, so I complimented her on the facility stating that it all sounds great, and asked her to go a little more in depth on certain topics to clarify a point she had already made despite the fact that she had done so perfectly the first time through. That was it, we said our goodbyes and I stated I was very interested and hope to hear from them soon. Less than an hour later I had an offer for the contract.

I was more than a little stunned on how fast this all happened, but thrilled at the same time. I now had two potential jobs lined up, and much to my surprise was not done yet. My phone rang again that afternoon and before I knew it interview two for the day was about to begin. It turned out that one of the facilities that I had told my first company to submit me to called out of nowhere. I had no advanced warning and was totally unprepared, more so than interview number one if you can believe it. The second interview happened in the same fashion as the first one with a man this time telling me about the facility, how they run it, and how I would fit into the picture. They again left time for questions at the end, which I elegantly fumbled my way through and that was it.

I immediately called the woman from the first company to let her know what happened. She became instantly apologetic stating that sometimes facilities do not give them warning and will call unannounced after a candidate has been submitted. She asked me how it went anyway and what I thought. I gave her my brief recount of our talk and we hung up. An hour later she told me I had the offer.

I went from having no job prospects fresh off passing my boards to three offers within a twenty-four hour period. There was travel company number one, who I had an offer with for an outpatient clinic in Virginia. There was the second travel company, whose offer would take me to an outpatient clinic right next to Chicago. Third then of course would be the permanent placement outpatient job near my home. Each job was looking for an answer by that Monday giving me one whole day to make a decision that was going to change my life. I had to make a decision.

Without too much hesitation I eliminated the offer from the first travel company. After seeing how nicely the process flowed and overall professionalism with the second travel company there was really no competition between the two. Now this brings us to our two options. It was my crossroads that life had laid in front of me, which could take me in two entirely different directions. Path number one as I saw it was my safe path that stood for a normal life, making alright money, had a reasonable commute, healthcare coverage, and simply doing life the way you are supposed to. It was a safe, smart, and secure position that I do not think many could have faulted me for. I could have justified it a million and one ways as to why this was just such a better decision that any sane person would take. On the other hand I had path number two. This choice stood for a career that I knew only the real bare bones of. It would make me leave not only my home, but my home state thrusting me out into the world to work at a clinic I had only seen on a map and with people I had never met for thirteen weeks. If you have read the title of this book you already know my decision, but allow me tell you why I chose the path of uncertainty.

Reason one was that I wanted to make more money plain and simple. I had substantial student loans (+$83,000), ideas of investing, amongst other things that I knew the $68,000 (~$50,000 after taxes!) was not going to take care of.

Reason two was to travel. Everyone thinks travel, especially extended travel, is for when you are older and reaching retirement age. Normal America today requires you to spend at least the first 20 years of your life getting an education, followed by 40 years of working and saving so that you can enjoy the last 20 years if you made enough money and are still able bodied enough. It is part of our society that I am not looking to take part of and this was a career path that gave me a way out. This opportunity would allow me explore an area that I have never seen for three months at a time. It would let me actually experience a location, through slow travel, as opposed to taking a week off from work to vacation and run through all the tourist attractions you can. This is important to me now, as I do not know what age forty, fifty, sixty, and beyond have in store or how healthy I may be then. As a healthcare provider you are on the front lines after traumatic events, and often see just how unpredictable life is through injuries, accidents, and other chance events no matter how much care you take of your own health. A career as a traveling physical therapist was giving me the option to avoid the deferred life plan of our country today. I wanted to live in new states, meet new people, and experience different environments for myself. This was also at the time when I was deciding if I wanted to live in my home state or move somewhere new to begin my life. The additional advantage of knowing you would be able to take as much or as little time off as you want in between contracts was a big draw as well. It seemed like the only career path that was going to provide me with the flexibility in life that I was in search of.

Reason three was because I thought it might make me better at my profession of physical therapy. It would give me a larger sample pool to learn from and decide if some of those advanced certifications are truly worth it. I was also not entirely convinced of which setting I wanted to work in at the time, as there were several I had yet to experience.

Reason four was because if I did not like it after the thirteen weeks, the full length of the contract, I could stop. There are no rules or obligations after your contract is finished unless you had previously agreed to it. You are not tied to anything. If this career path ended up not being for me I would just stop, go home three months later, and take a permanent job. This way I would have no regrets looking back, or any of those what if thoughts down the line. I would have given it a real try and made my own decision.

Now, that may have been a bit of a rant, but those were all the items floating around in my head that allowed me to make my decision. After accepting the contract everything else flowed perfectly. The clinic I was contracted to waited for me to get licensed, and I started working shortly thereafter. I also want to note what happened during my conversation with the permanent position that I turned down. When I declined their offer and told them the real reason why and the route I was going instead, the man who interviewed me actually sounded a bit excited for me. He was the first person to say now was the time if I ever was going to take that path. He insisted I let him know if I decide to come back. We have stayed in touch since.

That in a nutshell is how I went from graduating with my doctorate, taking and passing the boards, and began working as a traveling physical therapist. It was not as smooth as I initially thought it was going to be, but looking back it really could have been much worse. I hope that presented my journey to you in a more realistic and relatable way by showing you how the events actually unfolded.

Here is brief timeline of what has happened since that first assignment:

Timeline:

- Graduated in 2016 as a Physical Therapist with my doctorate
- Studied for the NPTE exam and passed the test on my first try in late July 2016
- Accepted my first contract that began on September 27th just outside of Chicago on the Indiana boarder where I found housing on the great lakes
- Contract number one was extended for an additional 13 weeks
- I took a month off of work to vacation with family overseas.
- Accepted contract number two, and road tripped from New Jersey to New Mexico
- Accepted contract number three in southern California
- Contract number three was extended for an additional 13 weeks
- I paid off all of my student loans!
- Took some time off to road trip the entire West Coast from San Diego to Oregon
- Accepted contract number four in Oregon where I wrote this book while overlooking the Columbia River and the state of Washington
- Extended contract number four for an additional 13 weeks
- To be continued...

Before we wrap this section up completely let me tell you I have made a ton of mistakes as a traveler. Almost all of these incidences happened early on in my travel career primarily through my first contract, the extension, and through the following contract. It was no ones fault but my own due to lack of knowledge in this field. Those mistakes literally cost me thousands upon thousands of dollars that I would have much rather seen get to my bank account. Since then I have remedied the situation by knowing my own worth, realizing what was negotiable in those contracts, learning how to extend contracts the right way, and the real questions you should be asking on the interview. This is the purpose of the blueprint in the following section, which I can confidently say will save you from suffering through the mistakes I have made. I truly hope this book helps you and takes out the learning curve that took me so long to grasp, and introduces you to a career with limitless opportunities.

Part Three: THE BLUEPRINT

Finally what you are really here for! Welcome to The Blueprint for new graduates. First of all, congratulations on making it this far and not being frightened away by any of the above content. Working as a traveling physical therapist was, and still is, truly the best career decision I could have made coming out of school despite my clear lack of knowledge about the profession. This section is where we will address the knowledge gaps and take it a step further. Upon completion you will know exactly how to go from passing your boards to getting that first assignment and beyond. The blueprint will cover the essentials including:

- Section 1: Choosing a company
- Section 2: Finding the right recruiter
- Section 3: Deciding on potential placements
- Section 4: Navigating the interview
- Section 5: After the interview
- Section 6: Housing, Packing, and Road Trips!

Shall we get started?

The Blueprint Section 1: Choosing a Company

The first step you need to decide on when pursing a career as a traveling healthcare professional is what company you will be partnering with on this journey. At this time in the market it will not be hard to find several that you see as potential candidates. As you read in my story I started out with one company who I thought would be a good fit for me, but quickly found out another company was more suited to my tastes. I discovered this through trial and error, and while I may gotten a few things right, mainly by accident, I will show you that there is a better way to go about this by prioritizing other more important factors before ultimately making your decision.

Let us begin with the obvious. How do you find out and learn about different companies? A good way to start is to ask other travelers if you are lucky enough to know of any. I would guess that you likely do not, but if you happen to do so then be sure to take advantage of that situation. If you are still in school ask your faculty if they know any travelers that they could put you in contact with. I would not ask them about choosing this as a career path, but to use them more so as a networking tool to expand your reach. If you still do not have any luck then get online and search through various social media groups. You will notice a trend of which companies to stay away from and others who get recommended routinely. I would not use any of the above steps as your ultimate decision maker, but merely to gain footing as a starting point in order to organize a list of potential options. No matter which company you decide on you will be able to find glowing reviews that state so-and-so company is the best thing in the world, and they are the only one I will ever work for followed by another reviewer who says they are an evil corporation with whom they would never do business with again after traveling halfway across the country only to find out they had a cancelled contract. Moral of the story here is to look for others as guidance as you begin, but you should always do your own due diligence and research.

Once you have accumulated your initial list it is time to do some digging. Start with each companies social media presence, and website to get as much information and data on them as possible. You might be able to pick up important clues when deciding if they are right for you in the comments section from other posters, as well as seeing how well run their online presence is. It is almost inexcusable for any major company nowadays to not have a decent website with a social media on multiple platforms. If a company seems to be lacking in this department I would not count them completely out, but move forward with the ones who seem more established. Also, there are plenty of travel healthcare professional social media groups that I would access to ask questions. These groups are full of friendly travelers who will point you in the right direction or answer any remaining questions you have. A lot of beginner questions have been answered before so by searching through a group's older posts you may discover just what you are looking for. Something that may be a notable concern here is to be careful with who responds to you if you decide to go ask questions through social media groups. Some companies have been known to monitor groups with fake profiles and try to recruit you to their company for obvious selfish reasons.

While the above steps will get you started and put you in the game there is still much more you need to know. The real truth about companies is that as far as getting and securing you contracts the company you choose is not the most important decision you will have to make. This is for several reasons. The first being almost all companies have access to the same contracts. Some companies claim to have, "exclusive contracts," but I have been offered these so called exclusive positions from a separate competing company as well therefore I do not recommend putting too much stock into those claims. The second reason is that the vast majority of companies will cover the same areas across the USA. If you are looking for a job in California, for example, any company will do and you will not need a specific one to find an assignment there. I have found this to be true for just about any state including Alaska and Hawaii. Again, all major companies for the most part have the same lists of potential positions that you will be able to apply for, it is more so a matter of timing regarding your contract dates, and having an honest recruiter who presents you with all available options. Your start and end working dates will ultimately put you in prime position for both contracts and interviews. When choosing a company make sure you talk to several and interview them on why you should choose them. They need to sell themselves to you not the other way around.

Once you have narrowed down your list of potential companies you can now begin contacting them. Things to look for when first contacting a company are if their responses to your questions come in a timely manner. This is very important! If some are slow to respond to you or are giving vague answers to any specific questions you ask then I would thank them for their time and move on. In this career where things can happen very quickly, and you can go from not having an assignment or any idea where you'll be working to getting ready to drive two states away on a few weeks notice you will want people on your side who do not leave anything up in the air. You are looking for prompt replies to any emails, phone calls or texts. There is also the complete opposite scenario where the company you have been interviewing is feeling too pushy and trying to rush you into contracts that you are unsure of without giving it time for proper thought. I would eliminate that option almost immediately as well. In the world of travel therapy it is not the end of the world saying no to a contract even though you may be wondering if it is the right decision at the time. You will have many other opportunities that come up so fast you will forget those decisions and be back on your travels in short order. Do not let anyone pressure you into signing anything.

Overall while I have my favorite companies that I choose to work with, the main reason I stick with one or two is because of the relationship I built with the recruiter or representative that I am in contact with, but we will get into this more in the next section. Remember, choosing one company over another in regards to potential contract placements or locations available is not a make or break decision. There are however absolutely other reasons to pick one company over the next. Let's take a closer look at what benefits one company may have over another and how you should truly base this decision.

The Pay Structure: Pay structure does vary from company to company in a sense. With all companies you will receive your hourly rate, a housing stipend, and a meal stipend so no complaints there. The difference is that some like to give you an extremely low hourly rate while maximizing stipends. I have personally seen contracts offering as little as $9 an hour. Others will go the opposite route and give you the industry standard in hourly pay for an area while keeping the stipends more reasonable. You should feel comfortable with how your pay is set up and for many this means avoiding extremes at either end. Now, having a lower hourly rate does mean an increase in non-taxed stipends and an increase in overall weekly net pay, which is tempting to many, but I would still ere on the

40

side of caution. Many, including myself, avoid the extremely low hourly rates for fear of drawing attention to you in case of an audit during tax time. I honestly do not know if this is true as I am not a tax professional, but it would certainly seem like a red flag for me that any healthcare provider is earning $9/hour. I recommended that you should keep your hourly wage in the mid $20s. Risk what you will at your own peril.

Licensing: This is a big one for me! Who is in charge of licensing? Being a travel therapist is great because it allows you to travel the country and see new and interesting places from deserts to beaches to mountains and forests. The downside is these new places often bring you to new state where you will have to get a new PT license. This is a pain no matter how you look at it because it can take both your time and money. I can speak from a physical therapists point of view and say that some states such as Oregon will have you licensed in two weeks, but others such as California or New Jersey take it to a new level for lag time of roughly three months. What you want to know from the company is how will the licensing be handled. Will you be on your own for it, or will they take care of it? You want to know if you are on your own to acquire the license will you then be reimbursed for the costs of everything required for it? This can include, but is not limited to, the application itself, fingerprints, background checks, medical screens, and specific continuing education credits to name a few. I will tell you this, applying for licenses and getting new licenses can be a huge headache and I would strongly recommend a company who takes care of this step for you and covers the complete costs.

Continuing Education: This is a necessary part of the medical healthcare field no matter what state you work in. What you want to know here is will the company pay for your continuing education or, once again, are you all on your own? As a traveler you will undoubtedly accumulate licenses based on how long you decide to pursue this career. I already have seven of them in my two years of work. While some states continuing education requirements for license renewal are simple and easy to achieve, others can be a bit more of a challenge. This may not seem like a big deal early on and certainly was the last thing on my mind when starting out traveling, but having access to free CEUs or a reimbursement plan for them through your company is a great advantage to have. Definitely take the time to find out how the company will handle this required aspect of your career.

Where am I going to live? Housing is another aspect that is generally similar between companies, but still it can vary. Typically you can take the housing stipend offered or allow the company to find you a place to live. It is highly recommended that you take the stipend! This is due to the fact that it puts you in charge of where you live, the cost for it, and any money you do not use is then yours to keep. It lets you decide how lavishly or frugally you want to live. There are times where it can be a large stress reliever to have your company take this step for you and many will do just that for their first contract to simplify the process even further. Also, some areas are just plain difficult to find housing and it can be easier to pass on the burden. I have always taken the stipend since the beginning and have never had an issue finding suitable and safe housing. Another benefit of the company having specific individuals who handle housing is that since contracts are often repeated by travelers within the same company they may be able to put you into contact with previous employees to ask where they stayed during their time at a certain location.

Retirement plans: 401k options and other retirement plans may or may not be offered through your travel company. Some companies have great 401k plans with a lot of options while others are limited or work with a third party that may have high fees or investments that you are not interested in. It is a good idea to look into this before you decide on a company if it is of interest to you. A very important aspect here is that some companies have an employer match for retirement accounts while others do not. This is something I took into consideration when looking into travel companies, but this step can also be tricky and not quite as straightforward as it seems. Many companies will say they absolutely have a company match, but then after some research you will realize they have a tiered approach to it. This basically means they will only match a certain percent after a full year of work. This percent will then go up for year two, three, etc. If you work with multiple companies this becomes challenging and you may never reach a full, or any, match on investments. Again this might not be a concern for you now, but if you plan on doing this for multiple years it may be something worth looking into.

Health insurance: This is often another important consideration for individuals and families alike. I have found through my experience that all companies do offer some form of health insurance, and I personally take my travel company's health insurance, however not all of these plans are created equal. Take a good look at the health insurance plans before deciding on if it will meet the needs for you and your family. This consideration will vary from person to person, and what you need to prioritize may be unique to you. This is especially true if you have a certain medical condition or are routinely sick. You always have the option to acquire your own health insurance independently. Additionally, you may lose healthcare coverage if you take extended absences between contracts so be sure to read the fine print and plan accordingly.

To summarize this section you need to ask around, but do your own research on companies to narrow down a list of who the winners might be for you. Once this is done remember that choosing a company for access to contracts is not what you should be prioritizing. Almost all the big players pool from the same list and have access to the same areas. What is more important is that you feel comfortable talking with whoever answers that phone for you and if they respond to you in a timely manner. As listed above the pay structure, licensing process, continuing education, housing, retirement planning, and health insurance are your real decisions here. There are other factors you may add to the list, but by prioritizing through these steps you will start out on the correct path for success.

The Blueprint Section 2: Finding the Right Recruiter

Choosing your recruiter is perhaps the most impactful decision you will have to make when beginning a traveling career. This is a very important step for many reasons, and if you can start your career off with the right recruiter on your side it will make a world of difference. Here we will take a moment to realize why this is such a critical step in our process.

To begin with, your recruiter is the main point of contact you will have with a travel company so it is imperative to get this correct from the get go. They are responsible for providing you with the potential list of assignment options including state, setting, and start time you desire. They are going to be the ones who present you to the various clinics, hospitals, and practices as a worthy candidate of consideration for contracts. It is through them you will make any changes or negotiations in your contract, which we will be discussing shortly in upcoming sections. If, for example, you are getting ready for an assignment and are in need of assistance with housing you will talk to them first and they will put you in contact with the appropriate person to come to your aid. If your assignment is not exactly as described in the contract you will bring this to their attention first. If you are not comfortable in a clinical setting for various reasons including, but not limited to, ethical decisions, fraudulent billing, or any other deviations from a contract they are your first point of contact. This is why it is essential to find a person who is the right fit for you and why we will utilize an entire section of our blueprint to identify the best way to complete this step.

In similar fashion as when selecting a company, step one is to find a recruiter that is quick to respond to you when you need to communicate anything to him or her. This can be a question, inquiry, or really anything at all that may come up. You are looking for very fast replies during workdays, but even after hours or on weekends you should have no problem getting a hold of them. Response time is a great gauge to decide if your current recruiter is suitable for your needs. You also want someone who will communicate with you in a way that is most comfortable and preferable to you. This could be phone calls, texts, or emails. I, for example, primarily am in contact with my recruiter through texts however we will also talk on the phone and email on occasion or as needed. This is important because when searching for a new assignment, negotiating a variety of factors within contracts, or accepting the assignment I am in constant contact with my recruiter. This dynamic immediately changes once I am on assignment however, and our conversations drop down to once a month. The rapport you build should be comfortable and not have any unnecessary tension. You are working together for a common goal, which is to get you on an assignment!

Qualities that should absolutely be avoided in a recruiter of course include anyone who feels aggressive or is too pushy about you taking an assignment. No one is to force you into a contract when you are unsure. You may feel this way due to an assignment's location, working in a setting you are not particularly familiar with or interested in, an overwhelming caseload that you learn about during the interview, or for any other reason that gives you pause. Anyone who is trying to rush and pressure you into a contract is not on your team and not someone you want representing you. There will always be more contracts and opportunities in this career path, and if you pass one up several more are just around the corner.

What are the best ways to find a recruiter whose abilities and personality suit you? Similar to finding a company the best option is to simply ask around especially if you are lucky enough to know of any travelers. If you do not know any travelers and do not have access to them through your social network then it is time to get on social media such and find groups there to begin your search. I have found that almost anyone will give you the name and number of their recruiter along with some honest thoughts about him or her. You should be wary of anyone who goes overboard when referring you to his or her recruiter though. This is because every company offers a referral bonus once a new traveler signs on and completes a full contract. This typically can be around $1,000, which is not exactly small change. If you are going to use someone as a referral make sure they can give you detailed information about their recruiter. Avoid those who state something like, "oh they're great and always get me the most money, work the least..." etc. Ultimately it is still best to try and use someone you know in real life and not online for an honest assessment. As always it is up to you to interview the recruiter and not rely on information from others. Interview several candidates who you have heard good things about and narrow down your list from there based on your conversations. You always have the option to change your representative in the future once a contract has ended even if you decide to stay with the same company.

Another decision you have to make through this process is if you will be working with primarily one recruiter or multiple recruiters from different companies. There are a couple schools of thought on this and I will present you the advantages and disadvantages to both. Some like the strategy of utilizing multiple recruiters through different companies as they believe it casts a bigger net when searching for your next contract, and may help you negotiate pay by creating competition around you. The drawbacks here is that it is definitely more to manage, more paperwork for you in the end, and potentially the feeling that a recruiter does not prioritize you as they know you may not take the contract with them in the end despite their effort. The benefits of working with one recruiter and company are that it simplifies and streamlines the process for you including the paperwork, licensing and reimbursement, and the potential relationship you may build with that one recruiter. The drawbacks are there is a possibility you may miss out on some potential money as recruiters compete for you. Personally, I did my real homework after my first contract extension and found a recruiter and company that meet all my needs and it is what I would recommend for any new graduate starting this profession. As you become more comfortable in the travel field I would encourage you to branch out to other companies, however for new graduates the easier you can make this process the better off you will be. I routinely am in talks with other companies and recruiters when beginning the search for my next assignment though to make sure I have a complete list of potential jobs in the state and setting I am interested in. Ideally if you can find the right recruiter for you I would go with that route. If you are unsure due to inconsistency, trouble contacting them or getting answers, or feelings of being pressured into contracts then I would recommend reaching out to others in search of a better fit for your situation.

In summary, you should begin by finding recommendations from real people if you are fortunate enough to know any travelers, and if not get online and obtain a handful of suggestions with whom you can begin your search with. Next take the time to call up these companies or get in contact with a specific recruiter to discuss your situation and interview them as they will be largely present in your future if you decide to work with them. Do not just choose a recruiter because someone recommended them to you with a few kind words. The best recruiter for one person may not be best suited for you due to a variety of reasons. Some may prefer a more hands off approach while others like to be in constant contact. Others may prefer different contact methods such as phone calls, texts, emails, etc. All of these may be a deciding factor for you and may sway you in one direction. Take your time with this step until you believe you have found the right one. Let a recruiter know if you want to prioritize specific locations, certain settings, or total compensation so they can keep your goals in mind as you search for contracts. For new graduates I recommend to begin this journey with one recruiter from one company. Once you are comfortable in your new profession then start to explore the idea of utilizing multiple representatives.

The Blueprint Section 3: Deciding Where to Work

At this point you have found a company that meets your needs using criteria in section one to narrow down your search while eliminating the options that do not fit your requirements. You have also had a chance to interview multiple recruiters and decide who is going to best represent you in a way that you are both confident, and comfortable with. This is the time where you can now move forward securely, and begin actually searching for your first assignment. In this section we will determine where you would like to submit for potential contracts.

First things first, what state do you want to work in? Now some of you may know exactly what state you want to work in, which makes it a straightforward process to find all available positions in that area. Others may have several states they may be interested in and are open to hearing the opportunities available in each. A third category we can include would be an individual open to an assignment in any state. A universal truth in the travel world, especially from a physical therapy perspective, is that the more specific you are about location, the more open you need to be about what setting you would like to work in. The opposite holds true as well meaning if you only want to work in private outpatient practices you will not be able to be as picky about where they are located. Neither of the above statements means it is impossible to find the exact location and setting you want, but know it will be much harder to come by. Regardless the process will be comparable and you will repeat the next several steps for any new state you want to incorporate.

To begin this process you will inform your recruiter of the state or states you would prefer to begin searching for jobs in. They may ask you at this time if you have a specific start date in mind. Back in my story I chose assignments that would begin when my summer job ended. You can specify either an exact date, give a general estimate that may span a couple weeks to a whole month, or simply state that you are open to the idea of all dates. Asking for the latter will give you the most options ranging from assignments starting within a few days to others that may be several weeks away.

With this information in hand your recruiter will present you with a list of potential assignments that meet, or are within acceptable deviations from the information you provided. The following is from a physical therapy outlook again as we have quite a few options regarding settings we are able to work in compared to other professions that may be a bit more limited. The response from your recruiter will typically come through email, and hopefully be quite lengthy. The list you will be able to see generally includes only the basics including the city, state, start date, and setting of the facility. I personally like to ask for a list that contains all settings despite the fact that I know I am really only considering one or two work environments. I do this because if there is a specific location that comes up that I am very interested in exploring I may sacrifice the setting I originally wanted to accommodate. Also, it is relatively easy to narrow down the complete list yourself.

After giving the list a good once over, and noting several that may be of greater interest to you it is then time to investigate the locations in which the assignments are available. I routinely go through a checklist utilizing tools from several websites when deciding if a location is truly right for me. First, I get on maps to see where it is located and the population of the city. Next I look at the surrounding landscape for areas of interest, which for me may be a national park or a nearby city. After that I check the crime rates, and livability scores of an area that can easily be found on numerous websites online. Other factors that routinely come up and may sway a decision are if family and friends are in the area, or within driving distance from a potential location. After making your way through that checklist you will be able to make an educated decision if an area is acceptable to you. Once your decision has been made you will relay that information to your recruiter who will proceed by presenting you to the clinics as a potential candidate. Once this is complete you will be playing the waiting game while the facility determines if they are interested in interviewing you for the position. Nothing at this point is official in any way so present to as many, or as few open contracts as you would like. It is generally a good idea to submit to all that you have a definite interest in as well as ones that you think might be reasonable. You can always turn down an offer later on if you determine it does not meet your needs. New graduates who are just beginning the job search are encouraged to apply to as many jobs as possible. It will give you practice for both researching new areas, and for future phone interviews.

If interested in working in multiple states you would simply repeat the above process for each state on your list. This is more than fine to do, and will allow you a glimpse of the job market for different locations. The only problems that may arise will be if you are not yet licensed in a specific state. Many contracts are looking for people with starting dates in the very near future therefore if you already have the state's license this will be a big advantage over other candidates. This does not always hold true as jobs can be posted several months out giving you the time necessary to get licensed. Other contracts, if they feel you are the right candidate for them, will often hold the position and wait for you to get licensed as well. One more thing of importance here is that some states will get you licensed faster than others. This can range from two weeks to three months in my experience depending on the state. Your company and recruiter will have the knowledge to help out here by providing realistic time frames through their previous travelers.

Once you have been submitted for the assignments of interest to you then your work is done. You will likely be in constant contact with your recruiter at this time because both of you are waiting on updates. During this short lived reprieve you can wait idly for the responses to see if you are selected for an interview, begin looking at new states for potential contracts if you have not done so already, or keep an eye on the current state where you have been searching in case a new opportunity comes along. New opportunities will present themselves often on a weekly basis so be prepared as a more enticing option may be right around the corner.

If a company thinks you are a practical candidate for them they will contact your recruiter who will then communicate the information to you. Your recruiter will inquire as to what hours you are available for a phone interview, or they may give you a selection of times and dates the representative for the facility is available. With this knowledge you will work together to find a time and date that works for both parties. Generally your recruiter will provide you the name of the person who will be calling to interview you, the company name, some information about the setting and place of work, and potentially the pay package if they have not done so already. Different companies withhold pay packages and present them to you at different times, but you can always request to know it up front. After that you are ready to interview for your first potential contract!

It is worth reaffirming that not every facility you submit to will interview you. This is based on a variety of factors including, but not limited to, experience in that setting and as a healthcare provider, available start date, or perhaps because they have accepted another candidate already. These contracts can be taken fast! Remember, you are competing for these potential placements against other travelers just as in any other job interview.

The Blueprint Section 4: Navigating the Phone Interview

It is now time for us to take a more in depth look at the phone interview. Your presentation here is a deciding step toward your first potential contract so it is critical to make the most of it. Through your recruiter you already know the date, time, and who will be calling you for the interview. Make sure you are set up at least ten minutes ahead of time in a nice quiet area with good phone reception and no distracting background noises. This is the first, and likely only, chance you will have to feel out a potential placement, present yourself professionally, ask any questions you have, and ultimately decide if an assignment is both a proper fit for you and one that you will be happy with for thirteen weeks.

The phone interview often will make first time travelers nervous as to many it sounds like an intense and daunting experience. I can happily tell you that those jitters are hardly warranted. The interviews themselves are actually relatively easy to navigate once you discover that they all follow a similar format, and can be broken down into three phases. Phase one is the introduction where all your basic pleasantries are expressed and some light chatting takes place as each party feels the other out. Phase two is the sell where you will be told all about the facility and how you will fit into their system. Interviewers can either get very in depth in this section, or you may notice them trying to quickly gloss over a few details. Phase three is time for your questions. This will be your only chance to attain the data needed to make an informed decision about an assignment, therefore we need to plan appropriately. It is time for us to break down these three phases.

Phase One: The interview will begin with the normal introductions as all on the line will introduce themselves. I say all for a reason. The vast majority of the time you will be on the phone with one other person, however this may not always be the case. There have been two separate instances where I have been interviewed in different formats to this. Once I was on speakerphone with three people on the other side, and a second time I was on the phone with one person but was told there was a second person from the department listening in. I tell you this because I had no idea these surprises could happen until they did. Do not let either of these throw you off your game, or allow others to overly control the conversation. Most importantly do not be intimidated, and shy away from any questions you have at the end.

Phase Two: Once all pleasantries and introductions have been exchanged, the interviewer will begin what I call the sell portion of the interview. This can be quite in depth or a simple narrative description of the facility, which I alluded to earlier. You are hoping for the former with as much information as you could possibly handle about a facility. You are about to start a job, sight unseen, so the more you know the better. A typical sell will include a description of the facility, plenty of information such as the number of other healthcare workers employed as staff, available assistants, equipment they have available, hours of operation, parking areas, and any other aspects they deem important. They may use this time to say anything about unique treatment options they provide as well. Next they will go through your typical day including: caseload expectations, paperwork time, specific patient populations they cater to, and how the documentation system works at their facility. Finally, they will conclude with what is expected from you coming in, and they may ask questions about your experience with various populations, treatment techniques, or information regarding your resume. Be ready with some paper and a pen handy here to jot down the important information, or any clarifications that will be needed for your questions in the next section.

Phase Three: The sell has come to an end and now it is your turn. They will begin by trying to gauge your interest level by asking your thoughts on the facility, and if it sounds like a place you would be interested in working. Next they will ask if you have any questions. The short answer is yes; you always have questions for them. Begin your questions with anything they have said so far that you would like clarification on from the notes you have already taken. Do not let any of their answers be left in vague terms as you are looking for specifics here. You want concrete numbers whether it is about the caseload you will be treating, or documenting time that is built into the day. Next you will go through your list of questions. It is highly recommend for you to have your additional questions written down beforehand in a checklist manner to make things as efficient as possible. If questions were answered in the prior sections just write down the information as the interview progresses. Below is a list I have compiled for my need to know information that must be answered if I am considering an assignment. It is likely that during the sell portion about half of these will already have answers. The remaining information will be up to you to uncover.

Need to Know Questions List:
- When is the start date?
- What is the daily schedule/how many patients will I see per day? i.e. caseload
- How much time do I have per patient treatment and evaluation?
- Does this position guarantee 40 hours per week?
- Are there any weekends required to work? Or is overtime available?
- What documentation system do you use?
- How much time will I have for orientation and what will that look like?
- How will I be documenting? Is it electronic, written, or dictation? Do I have my own device or station to work at?
- How many other therapists are on staff? PT, OT, ST, assistants or aides?
- Will I be supervising anyone?

- What equipment do you have available at your facility? Are private treatment rooms available?
- What hours will I be working? Are these flexible?
- Is there documentation time built into the day?
- Is there a lunch break, if so what time and how long?
- Why is there a need for a traveler at your facility?

This is a great general list that will cover all of your bases, and give you the information needed to come to a proper conclusion. If you can get these questions answered it will provide a strong understanding of the facility as well as what a typical day of work will look like. These questions are extremely important for a future reason. If the contract is offered to me that I ultimately accept, I will have my recruiter put the answers to several of these questions directly into the contract. If it is not written down it does not exist. The main three I specifically ask to be written into the contract include the caseload I will see per day, the time per patient treatment and the time per patient evaluation, and any promised documenting time built into the day. There are some bad stories out there of travelers who are taken advantage of and I do not want you to be one of them. Having those three in writing basically blocks your day out so no surprises may be added in there. Anything else that is of importance to you needs to be in writing.

Overall, the interview itself is a relatively quick affair with most averaging twenty minutes or less. Again, this is likely the only opportunity you will have to get your questions answered before an official offer is made. Be sure to come prepared and ready to make good use of your time.

The Blueprint Section 5: After the Interview

Congratulations on completing your first phone interview and being one step closer to securing your first contact! Not only did you do it with proper planning, but also with the foresight and knowledge of what exactly was coming at you. In doing so you were able to ask the must know questions, and gathered all the data necessary to make an informed decision on whether this location will be suitable for you. After completing your interview the next step will be to notify your recruiter. He or she will often ask you how you feel it went, and your overall thoughts on the placement to gauge your interest. Feel free to tell them as much, or as little as you want at this point. It is likely that if you were selected for the interview the facility already has a strong interest in you, and there will likely be an offer coming your way shortly assuming there were no hiccups during the phone call. I can honestly say that I have gotten an offer after every interview I have participated in, and this includes my first contract as a brand new graduate. After speaking with other travelers I have met on the road it appears most have had similar experiences. I tell you this so that you are prepared for what is next as it is very common practice for a facility to make an official offer that same day. I have had an offer presented to me as quickly as an hour after the completion of the interview. The less likely situation is that there is no offer. If that is the case you simply continue with the steps from the previous sections until you reach this stage.

Once you have received an offer your short window of opportunity is open. At this point you have all the information needed as well as the pay package. It is up to you whether you are ready to accept, decline, or attempt to negotiate any aspect of what was discussed. This is where I feel even the more experienced travelers drop the ball, and miss out on a chance to take control of several aspects of a contract. This can be due to a lack of knowledge, or for fear of negotiating. I tell all new graduates that everything in a contract is negotiable especially the hours and days you will be working, scheduled paperwork time, and the pay package. Once an offer is made the facility is looking for a quick reply, within twenty-four hours typically, which does not give you an extended period of time to think and devise a strategy on what you would like to negotiate. Due to the timeframe it is best to focus on just a few key areas that you may want to adjust or change. Remember, although you have received an official offer does not mean a facility will stop interviewing potential candidates, or putting out offers to others previously interviewed if you are dragging your feet. This is why the travel game is so fast, and if you do not take action the game will quickly pass you by. As you can see one can go from not having any ideas on where and when you will be working to all of a sudden packing for an assignment in the next state over. This spontaneity is what can also be a lot of fun, and I for one enjoy. You have a job and opportunity that can take you anywhere you want to see, explore, and put your clinical skills to good use. This job is part choice, part chance, and has the capability of taking you on adventures you never dreamed of.

We need to discuss what to, and what not to negotiate now. After my first contract as a new graduate where I missed out on thousands of dollars I can tell you I have never accepted a pay package that is initially offered to me. This is not out of greed, but I want fair compensation for the work I do. This makes it important to know your worth. There are multiple factors that can, and should be taken into account when negotiating a fair pay package. This includes the amount of work expected of you and caseload you will be handling, as well as the location and cost of living expenses in a particular area. One of the real benefits of traveling is the compensation over permanent positions so do not miss out here. I have talked to many other travelers about take home pay and what is considered on both the low and high ends of the spectrum. As a physical therapist, whether you are a new grad or experienced veteran, your weekly take home net pay should fall between $1,500-$1,700. I would never accept anything lower than that regardless of area, caseload, or setting, but I would absolutely expect higher compensations based on the same criteria. Imagine the differences in working in a more expensive such as San Francisco CA. The current housing market is clearly on the higher end, and I would expect to have a larger check at the end of the week because of it. With that in mind take a look at your pay package, the above information I have provided you with, and decide what is needed to make this assignment work for you. Taking your time will pay dividends, and grant you access to hundreds if not thousands of dollars over your contract length. Once you decide on a number you can inform your recruiter and you will wait for a reply. Do not be afraid to walk away from an assignment, as unfortunately this sometimes must be done.

Other aspects that I will routinely negotiate are the work schedule, and built in paperwork time. You will find some facilities more flexible than others in these regards. For example, I always prefer to work four ten-hour days. While most contracts do not offer this upfront it has routinely been accepted in my experience. I do this simply because I just moved to a brand new area and three day weekends make exploring the surrounding landscape much easier. Negotiating paperwork time into your schedule has been a hit or miss experience for me. It is worth the attempt as on several occasions I have been able to work a half hour of paperwork time into my schedule at the end of my days. This makes a workday flow much easier, and keeps stress levels to a minimum, as I know I will not fall behind with documenting time. What I do not try to negotiate is caseload. Facilities typically have requirements of how many patients their workers are to treat to meet a general quota. Instead of asking for more or less of a caseload, just make sure your compensation will reflect the amount of work you put in.

Before finalizing any contract make sure you read the fine print. All the routine things from schedule, pay package, and dress code amongst other things should be in there already. What you need to do here is get anything promised to you during the phone interview in writing. If you were told one hour time blocks for evaluations, and forty five minutes for treatments then this needs to be in there. This goes for paperwork time, lunch breaks, or anything else you may think is important. If they said it to you during the interview then this should be no problem. If it is a problem, and they are opposed to putting specific numbers in writing then decline and move on as they are looking to take unfair advantage of you. The contract is there not only as an agreement, but also as protection for both parties involved as well.

One important aspect of the contract that you need to find is the cancellation policy. All companies will provide this in writing, but what will vary is the amount of notice required. This is a very important clause that is not to be overlooked for your own security. Facilities can cancel contracts on travelers, and it does happen from time to time for various reasons. The most common reason for a cancelled contract is if a facility recently hired a new healthcare worker for the permanent position you were temporarily filling. These situations can happen so knowing the cancellation policy can better prepare you if these unfortunate events occur. Often times companies will offer two-week cancellation notices, as in they have to give you a full two-week notice before ending the contract. This is not enough time in my opinion. I recommend, and only sign contracts with thirty-day cancellation policies. This is because I often travel further distances for contracts in areas of the country I have yet to see. You do not want to arrive at a contract only to be given your two weeks notice after a several day road trip to get there. Add in the fact that you are in a brand new area that you are completely unfamiliar with far from family and friends can create an awful experience for any traveler. Thirty-day notices are also useful for housing as well because if you paid up front for the duration of your contract and it was cancelled after two weeks you just threw away a substantial amount in regards to rent. Thirty-day cancellation policies are the clear recommendation here.

The Blueprint Section 6: Housing, Packing, and Road Trips!

Welcome to the final section of the blueprint. By using the advice from the previous sections you have set yourself up for success as a traveling healthcare provider. At this point you have completed all the steps necessary to ensure you are partnered with a company and representative that have your best interests in mind, are traveling to an area you have researched and have chosen to be of interest for you, will be working in a setting that you are comfortable with, and have created an solid contract that not only protects you, but is also more lucrative than any permanent position you may have otherwise found. Typically, once the contract is signed, people have one of two reactions, or sometimes a combination of both. You are either beyond excited to begin your new adventurous career, or are wondering if this was the right decision compared to the, "safe plan," that all of your peers will be taking. No matter how you are feeling at this time remember that contracts are short lived. Once your thirteen weeks are completed you are absolutely in no way obligated to continue with this career path if you decide it is not for you. In the absolute worst-case scenario it was a great learning experience where you built a great financial base and were able to see a new part of the world. At best it is the only career you will ever know because of the long list of benefits I have talked about in previous sections.

Now that the contract is signed there are several more steps you will have to take before you begin working. I call these the three hurdles and break them down in this section. The hurdles include: finding suitable housing, packing, and the road trip. While there are many ways to go about these steps I will give you my recommendations from personal experience and conversations with other travelers. These final steps can be as easy or hard as you make them out to be.

Hurdle 1: Finding Housing

One of the biggest challenges of being a traveler is finding housing in the area you will soon be calling home for the next several months. To this day finding housing is always a concern of mine, however it is also one that somehow works out perfectly in the end regardless of my worries. This is never more true than right now as I write this section of the book in a rented a house on the Oregon coast staring at the Pacific Ocean. The house itself is fully furnished with access to laundry, Internet, and everything else you could hope for at only $700 per month. Now not all of my previous housing options have turned out to be quite as nice as this, but the more I travel the better I get at finding these options. I will give you my advice on how best to go about finding housing in safe areas, and the resources I rely on.

My process for the first two assignments I had taken began by finding the location of where I will be working on Google maps. Next I would search all the nearby areas for apartment complexes that had solid reviews with written verbal feedback. I would make a list and then call up every single one of them up to find out if they would do a 13-week stay, or month to month rent. This was either met with a prompt yes or no, which quickly narrowed down my search results. To all those who said yes I would then ask for the price, and what's included in the unit. At the time I was simply looking for a kitchen with basic appliances, and a washer and dryer in unit or on the premises. You can always ask if an apartment complex offers furnished units, as many will at an increased rate. This option, despite the price, may be worth it to you as a new traveler, and will ensure you have everything needed. The above process got me through my first several assignments. I stayed in unfurnished units, put down an air mattress, bought a small portable card table, and became what I called home. It was a bit of a spartan existence and definitely not for everyone, but I knew the area I chose and how little time I was actually going to be spending in the apartment. I was also fresh out of school and used to living a minimalistic lifestyle. Overall, I enjoyed utilizing apartment complexes early on as they can function as their own little community in a city that I was otherwise unfamiliar with. This potentially saved me from choosing a bad area on the wrong side of town.

For my next assignments I switched from the unfurnished units, and apartment complexes to utilizing Airbnb and VRBO. This time around I was able to find furnished houses with all the creature comforts you could ask for. Not only was finding housing much cheaper this way since the hosts were flexible in all aspects, but I also felt very spoiled after living in the unfurnished units. I discovered that often times if you contact the host and let them know you are a traveling medical professional coming to the area for work on a contract they become very willing to work out a deal. It not only lets them know you can afford the monthly rental price, but also that you are a professional who is not going to cause chaos in their home.

My current assignment that I alluded to earlier, where I am currently watching the waves crashing on the beach, is the first assignment I have used Craigslist in combination with a local realtor to find housing. Again, it is a fully furnished house with everything you could possibly need. I, like many travelers, was hesitant at first about using Craigslist because there had been a lot of noise regarding more scams on this medium versus any others for finding housing, but it turned out great. It has easily been the best combination of value and price I have found since beginning my traveling journey. I took an extra step here though as I found and called a local realtor who was able to confirm the listing for me as they knew the owners. It turned out it was their summer home so they were looking to create a side hustle by renting it in the off-season.

Other options for fellow travelers include social media groups for renters in a certain area. I have yet to go that route personally and for that reason I will hold off on my recommendations. At the very least it is another option others have used successfully, and may give you a good lead on where to start your housing search. You always have the option of having roommates as well, but I have always stuck with having my own place and recommend you do the same. For your first assignment you want to control as many variables as possible to streamline the process and a difficult roommate can absolutely derail an otherwise great situation. As you can see there are various options and one of the above ways is bound to find you a suitable home for your stay, just make sure you pick a safe area! If worst comes to worst, and this step is causing too much stress then simply have your travel company set it up for you.

One last topic to touch on before moving on is monthly rent. Many new travelers have asked me how much they should really be spending on rent. This is very common because a lot of new graduates either commuted or lived on campus, and may not have had too much experience with this aspect of life yet. Regardless of area I would recommend that rent should be less than 1 week of your take home pay. This is a good place to start for many, but ultimately it is up to you and your budget. When I began traveling my goal was to pay off my student loans as fast as possible, and therefore was looking to save as much as I could. As a result I often only spent half of my weekly take home pay here. It will take some research, negotiation, and a few phone calls, but I would expect and encourage you to aim for these amounts as well.

Hurdle 2: Packing

As I engage and guide more new graduates who are interested in pursuing this profession packing is always a question that, in time, never fails to be brought up. People are generally polarized in this aspect, and will fall toward one end of the spectrum. This means a futile attempt to pack their whole life into a vehicle, or taking the bare minimum needed to get by. It is not just new graduates who stumble on this as I have met seasoned travelers on both ends as well. I have known some who carry everything with them to live in an unfurnished apartment comfortably as well as others who pack golf clubs, snowboards, or bikes and then rely on finding furnished housing to cover the remaining essentials. The answer to this question in reality is entirely dependent upon you. Ideally you want to travel as light, but also as comfortable as possible. This generally means having the necessary essentials plus a few recreational items for you to enjoy without having your car overflowing to the point where you cannot see out of the windows. In a profession when you are potentially relocating every three months the easier you can make the transitions between assignments the simpler life will be. You will always have the ability and the means to acquire the missing items that repeatedly come up and would be useful for you to have as you travel.

Here is a quick rundown that may help you decide on what to bring. Start off with the essentials, which for most is the electronics that luckily do not take up much room. I have my laptop, e-reader, and all associated items with chargers in a backpack. Once this is squared away pack clothing you will need for work, followed by what is needed for recreational activities. Work clothes are often needed to comply with the dress code of a facility so do not go overboard here as your next assignment may require something else entirely. For example one contract may want you to wear a blue polo, black pants and tennis shoes while the next may want dress shirts and shoes. Many overestimate how much clothing will actually be needed on the road so pack light and pick up the rest as you go. The next thing to take into consideration is recreational equipment. This one may be decided, to an extent, on where your assignment is located. If you go somewhere that is near the mountains with plenty of snowboarding and skiing nearby for example, you would likely pack differently compared to a location near beaches. Odds are that wherever you go you will have the opportunity to rent, or if you are lucky borrow, the items needed for a weekend of fun here. This has happened to me several times where coworkers let me borrow snowboards, backpacks, camping equipment, bikes, and much more that allows me to travel lighter.

Additionally, I started out traveling with a fold up bed and a card table that I bought online in preparation for living in unfurnished apartments, but over the last year I have yet to use them as my housing has already been furnished. What happens now is I unpack my car and put them out of the way somewhere until it is time to load my car back up. While they were quite useful for my first empty apartment rentals I am now thinking of unloading them to free up space in my car. This same holds true for some of the kitchen items, and toiletries I began traveling with. If you are moving into furnished housing you will not have to worry about these kinds of items, and can start out with just the basics. When you arrive at your assignment you will quickly realize if you are missing any necessities, and can plan appropriately from there.

The above may come a lot easier to those who may have already been living this lifestyle since undergraduate, and are now professional car packers. Others may have a harder time struggling to fit their life into a small space. All travelers though will quickly come up with their own unique system to solving the car-packing dilemma.

Hurdle 3: Road Trip!

The third and final hurdle to get you and your freshly packed car to your new temporary housing is the road trip. The road trip is one part of traveling that has quickly become an adventure and vacation all in itself for me. While others may look at it in despair I strongly encourage you to take full advantage of the opportunity to plan this out, and make it as much fun as possible.

At this point in my travel career I have driven through two iconic USA road trip routes in their entirety. This includes the historic Route 66, which starts in Chicago and ends at the Santa Monica Pier in California, and the pacific coast highway with the addition of the entire Oregon coast from bottom to top. For me these have become some of my favorite memories since beginning my traveling career. There are countless stops, scenic viewpoints, and much more that you will find on the road if you do not rush the experience. Road trips allow you to see so much of the country while you travel for days, or even weeks at time so that when you finally reach your assignment you are ready to settle back in and return to your working ways. I have experienced more of the country in my relatively short time traveling than many will in their entire lives through proper planning of this step, and you can do the same.

I am sure there are multitudes of ways to plan a road trip, but I will tell you how I go about the process. Step one is to get on Google maps again, and find the most direct route to get to your assignment. You will often be presented with several viable options, which is great as one path may be of greater appeal to you for various reasons. Now you need to look along that route to discover if there are any areas that are worth spending time in. This will again vary from person to person dependent on what your idea of fun is. Some of my favorites to search for along the way are national and state parks, hiking trails, museums, botanical gardens, and any big city to get out and walk around in. I will often go out of my way on road trips for certain sites, or plan the whole trip based on one or two prime locations. I have most recently done this when I planned my last road trip around Yosemite National Park to spend extra days there. It was absolutely worth it!

Once you have decided on the stops you can then answer the next few questions that will come up with all road trip planning. The top two questions asked by new graduates refer to how much driving you should do in a day, and how to go about booking hotels or other means of lodging? Answering the former is difficult as I cannot tell you exactly what your specific driving limit should be as some may tolerate the miles on the road better than others. I can however guide you from my experience and what I have done in the past in regards to both aspects.

Early on when I started traveling I would drive up to eight hours a day with two planned stops to break up the drive, and stretch out the legs for an hour or two at a time. A typical day would have me waking up early, start driving for three to five hours to get to the first stop that may be a hike, museum, or park. I would take my time to explore the area, and then head back to the car to finish up the remainder of the drive or make it to the next planned stop. This worked just fine as it allowed me to travel to new areas quickly. The downfall of this routine was that I would often miss out on some sites or feel rushed because I was prioritizing trying to cover as much ground as possible during the daylight hours. I do not do this anymore as I have taken a more relaxed approach to travel. The most I drive now is six hours per day, but more often than not it is four to five hours per day on any given road trip. The decreased amount of time in the car is great and gives me much more freedom and time to explore areas in greater depth. It is what I recommend to all new travelers now.

Depending on how far you will be traveling you must do the math and take into consideration how many road trip days will be needed to reach your ultimate destination. I would advise everyone to arrive at a new location two days before your assignment begins. This is for you to get a lay of the land, find where to get groceries, and anything else you might need before you begin working. Start this process by planning your trip in reverse order from the day in which you would like to arrive, and working backwards through your stops until you have a full plan.

Next we need to cover lodging on the road. When I started traveling I would book everything up to three or four days in advance, which basically put myself on autopilot. This was nice as it made everything very easy and straightforward on where my endpoints for each day were. It streamlined the process, but still it was not without its limitations. I have since moved away from that method not because it did not work, but only to give myself greater freedom and flexibility on the road. Now I take everything one day at a time. How I do this process now is by booking my hotel or other lodging one-day in advance. A typical day would have me wake up and begin driving, making my stops, and arriving at my hotel typically before nightfall. Once in my hotel and winding down I then take a look at the next day, decide on how much I want to drive or how long I would like to spend in an area, and proceed to book my next hotel accordingly. I transitioned to this because some areas have quite a bit more to see than others. Other locations with less to offer I may opt to pass straight through while listening to a good audiobook. For the above reasons I recommend booking as you go.

There are several other tips and tricks that I have picked up while mapping out road trips that I would like to share with you. Choosing lodging that serves breakfast is a great option that can really simplify your morning. It is something I do almost exclusively now just to make the waking hours easier. Even if a hotel costs a little more the time you save with this is often worth it. Next take into account if you are driving into sunrise or sunset. It may not seem like a big deal now, but it certainly can be. I speak from experience on this one and it is no fun driving blinded by glare on a new and unfamiliar road with other cars speeding past you. Third, try to arrive before dark. Others may be more comfortable with this, but I am not a fan of driving through unfamiliar areas at night so I intentionally plan my road trips to arrive at the day's location before last light. Doing so provides me with ample time to wind down for that night. Finally, make sure you leave early. If the sun is up your should be to! There is plenty of time to sleep in when you get to your destination, but now is the time to explore. This may be your one and only chance to see a location as you are passing through. An extra bonus note is that podcasts, and audiobooks are your friend and should be used abundantly!

Drive safely friends.

Conclusion:

I truly hope this book has been helpful for you, and provides you with the guidance and bravery to start your career as a traveling healthcare provider. While it may be scary for some to start a career that you likely received no information about during your countless hours spent in the classroom, I really believe this is the best career path for a new graduate. If you want to get rid of your student loans while slow traveling the country and progressing your skills as a healthcare provider then this is the career for you. There is a world of adventure out there if you are willing to take advantage of it.

I would like to take this time to make a final offer to you. Since traveling I have personally worked with, and have spoken to countless recruiters and companies. In doing so I have acquired my own personal list of representatives who I would strongly recommend to any new graduate or seasoned travel veteran. These are the recruiters who have put me first and listened to how I wanted to prioritize my assignments in regards to pay, location, and setting. If you are interested in a further jumpstart to your journey with a tried and tested recruiter, and company behind you, you can email me at Dr.DelTufo@gmail.com. I will provide you with the name and number to reach out to, as well as answer any other questions you may have. I do not want you to take my word for it though. Utilize the steps in the appropriate sections to make sure anyone whom I recommend fits your specific needs. Do not be shy as traveling and discussing travel plans are some of my favorite topics!

Good luck and I hope to meet you on the road!

- Dr. Matthew Del Tufo PT, DPT

About the Author:

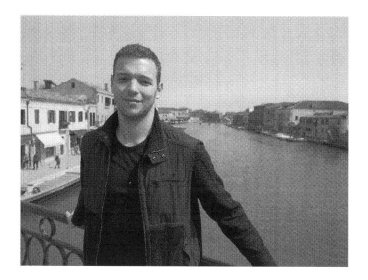

Dr. Matthew Del Tufo is a practicing Physical Therapist currently licensed in seven states across the country. He has pursued a career as a traveling Physical Therapist since graduating with his Doctorate from Stockton University in 2016.

Since graduating Dr. Del Tufo has coached and guided countless new graduates through the process of establishing their own careers in the traveling healthcare profession. Additionally, he provides private financial coaching services to help all new graduates combat the current student loan epidemic.

Made in the USA
Monee, IL
12 January 2020

20235929R10050